Delicious Vegan Cookbook

Budget Friendly Vegan Recipes Easy to Prepare at Home for Stay Healthy Increase Life and Losing Weight

Franck Renner

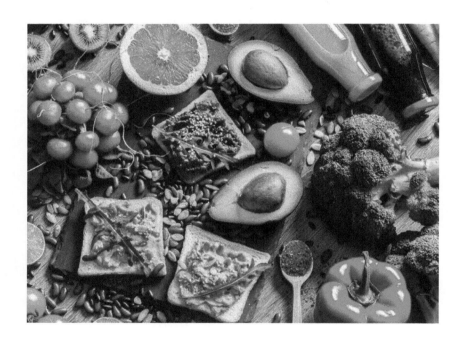

Table of Contents

copy and is only allowed with the express written consent from the Publisher. All additional right reserved.

The information in the following pages is broadly considered a truthful and accurate account of facts and as such, any inattention, use, or misuse of the information in question by the reader will render any resulting actions solely under their purview. There are no scenarios in which the publisher or the original author of this work can be in any fashion deemed liable for any hardship or damages that may befall them after undertaking information described herein.

Additionally, the information in the following pages is intended only for informational purposes and should thus be thought of as universal. As befitting its nature, it is presented without assurance regarding its prolonged validity or interim quality. Trademarks that are mentioned are done without written consent and can in no way be considered an endorsement from the trademark holder.

INTRODUCTION

The Merriam Webster Dictionary defines a vegetarian as one contains a wholly of vegetables, grains, nuts, fruits, and sometimes eggs or dairy products. It has also been described as a plant-based diet that relies wholly on plant-foods such as fruits, whole grains, herbs, vegetables, nuts, seeds, and spices. Whatever way you want to look at it, the reliance wholly on plants stands the vegetarian diet out from other types of diets. People become vegetarians for different reasons. Some take up this nutritional plan for medical or health reasons. For example, people suffering from cardiovascular diseases or who stand the risk of developing such diseases are usually advised to refrain from meat generally and focus on a plant-based diet, rich in fruits and vegetables. Some other individuals become vegetarians for religious or ethical reasons.

On this side of the spectrum are Hinduism, Jainism, Buddhism, Seventh-Day Adventists, and some other religions. It is believed that being a vegetarian is part of being holy and keeping with the ideals of non-violence. For ethical reasons, some animal rights activists are also vegetarians based on the belief that animals have rights and should not be slaughtered for food. Yet another set of persons become vegetarians based on food preference. Such individuals are naturally more disposed to a plant-based diet and find meat and other related food products less pleasurable. Some refrain from meat as a protest against climate change. This is based on the environmental concern that rearing livestock contributes to climate change and greenhouse gas emissions and the waste of natural resources in maintaining such livestock. People are usually very quick to throw words around without exactly knowing what a Vegetarian Diet means. In the same vein, the term "vegetarian" has become a popular one in recent years. What exactly does this word connote, and what does it not mean?

At its simplest, the word "vegetarian" refers to a person who refrains from eating meat, beef, pork, lard, chicken, or even fish. Depending on the kind of vegetarian it is, however, a vegetarian could either eat or exclude from his diet animal products. Animal products would refer to foods such as eggs, dairy products, and even honey! A vegetarian diet would, therefore, refer to the nutritional plan of the void of meat. It is the eating lifestyle of individuals who depend on plant-based foods for nutrition. It excludes animal products, particularly meat - a common denominator for all kinds of Vegetarians - from their diets. A vegetarian could also be defined as a meal plan that consists of foods coming majorly from plants to the exclusion of meat, poultry, and seafood.

This kind of Vegetarian diet usually contains no animal protein.

It is completely understandable from the discussion so far that the term "vegetarian" is more or less a blanket term covering different plant-based diets. While reliance majorly on plant foods is consistent in all the different types of vegetarians, they have some underlying differences. The different types of vegetarians are discussed below:

Veganism: This is undoubtedly the strictest type of vegetarian diet. Vegans exclude the any animal product. It goes as far as avoiding animal-derived ingredients contained in processed foods. Whether its meat, poultry products like eggs, dairy products inclusive of milk, honey, or even gelatin, they all are excluded from the vegans.

Some vegans go beyond nutrition and go as far as refusing to wear clothes that contain animal products. This means such vegans do not wear leather, wool, or silk.

Lacto-vegetarian: This kind of vegetarian excludes meat, fish, and poultry. However, it allows the inclusion of dairy products such as milk, yogurt, cheese, and butter. The hint is perhaps in the name since Lacto means milk in Latin.

Ovo-Vegetarian: Meat and dairy products are excluded under this diet, but eggs could be consumed. Ovo means egg.

Lacto-Ovo Vegetarian: This appears to be the hybrid of the Ovo Vegetarian and the Lacto-Vegetarian. This is the most famous type of vegetarian diet and is usually what comes to mind when people think of the Vegetarian. This type of Vegetarian bars all kinds of meat but allows for the consumption of eggs and dairy products.

Pollotarian: This vegetarian allows the consumption of chicken.

Pescatarian: This refers to the vegetarian that consumes fish. More people are beginning to subscribe to this kind of diet due to health reasons.

Flexitarian: Flexitarians are individuals who prefer plant-based foods to meat but have no problem eating meats once in a while. They are also referred to as semi-vegetarians.

Raw Vegan: This is also called the raw food and consists of a vegan that is yet to be processed and has also not been heated over 46 C. This kind of diet has its root in the belief that nutrients and minerals present in the plant diet are lost when cooked on temperature above 46 C and could also become harmful to the body.

Oatmeal Walnut Bread

Preparation Time: 15 minutes

Cooking Time: 1.5 hours

Serving Size: 1 ounce per serving

Ingredients:

- ¾ cup whole-wheat flour
- ¼ cup all-purpose flour
- ½ cup brown sugar
- 1/3 cup walnuts, chopped
- ¼ cup oatmeal
- ¼ teaspoon of baking soda
- Two tablespoons baking powder
- One teaspoon salt
- 1 cup Vegan buttermilk
- ¼ cup of vegetable oil
- Three tablespoons aquafaba

Direction:

1. Add into the bread pan the wet ingredients then followed by the dry ingredients.

2. Use the "Quick" or "Cake" setting of your bread machine.

3. Allow the cycles to be completed.

4. Take out the pan from the machine.

5. Wait for 10 minutes, then remove the bread from the pan.

6. Once the bread has cooled down, slice it and serve.

Nutrition: Calories: 80 | Carbohydrates: 11g Fat: 3g | Protein: 2g

Pumpkin Raisin Bread

Preparation Time: 15 minutes

Cooking Time: 1.5 hours

Serving Size: 1 ounce (28.3g)

Ingredients:

- ½ cup all-purpose flour
- ½ cup whole-wheat flour
- ½ cup pumpkin, mashed
- ½ cup raisins
- ¼ cup brown sugar
- Two tablespoons baking powder
- One teaspoon salt
- One teaspoon pumpkin pie spice
- ¼ teaspoon baking soda
- ¾ cup apple juice
- ¼ cup of vegetable oil
- Three tablespoons aquafaba

Direction:

1. Place all ingredients in the bread pan in this order: apple juice, pumpkin, oil, aquafaba,

---

flour, sugar, baking powder, baking soda, salt, pumpkin pie spice, and raisins.

2. Select the "Quick" or "Cake" mode of your bread machine.

3. Let the machine finish all cycles.

4. Remove the pan from the machine.

5. After 10 minutes, transfer the bread to a wire rack.

6. Slice the bread only when it has completely cooled down.

Nutrition: Calories: 70 | Carbohydrates: 12g Fat: 2g | Protein: 1g

Hawaiian Bread

Preparation Time: 10 minutes

Cooking Time: 3 hours

Serving Size: 1 ounce (56.7g)

Ingredients:

- 3 cups bread flour
- 2 ½ tablespoons brown sugar
- ¾ teaspoon salt
- Two teaspoons quick-rising yeast
- One egg
- ¾ cup pineapple juice
- Two tablespoons almond milk
- Two tablespoons vegetable oil

Direction:

1. Pour all wet ingredients first into the bread pan before adding the dry ingredients.
2. Set the bread machine to "Basic" or "Normal" mode with a light crust colour setting.

3. Allow the machine to finish the mixing, kneading, and baking cycles.

4. Take out the pan from the machine.

5. Transfer the bread to a wire rack.

6. After one hour, slice the bread and serve.

Nutrition: Calories: 169 | Carbohydrates: 30g Fat: 3g | Protein: 4g

Sweet Potato Bread

Preparation Time: 10 minutes

Cooking Time: 3 hours

Serving Size: 2 ounces (56.7g)

Ingredients:

- 4 cups bread flour
- 1 cup sweet potatoes, mashed
- ½ cup brown sugar
- Two teaspoons yeast
- 1 ½ teaspoon salt
- ½ teaspoon cinnamon
- ½ cup of water
- Two tablespoons vegetable oil
- One teaspoon vanilla extract

Direction:

1. Add the wet ingredients first, then follow by dry ingredients to the bread pan.
2. Use the "Normal" or "Basic" mode of the bread machine.

3. Select the light or medium crust colour setting.

4. Once the cycles are finished, take out the machine's bread, Cooldown the bread on a wire rack before slicing and serving.

Nutrition: Calories: 111 | Carbohydrates: 21g Fat: 2g | Protein: 3g

Black Forest Loaf

Preparation Time: 20 minutes

Cooking Time: 3 hours

Serving Size: 2 ounces (56.7g)

Ingredients:

- 1 ½ cups bread flour
- 1 cup whole wheat flour
- 1 cup rye flour
- Three tablespoons cocoa
- One tablespoon caraway seeds
- Two teaspoons yeast
- 1 ½ teaspoons salt
- One ¼ cups water
- 1/3 cup molasses
- 1 ½ tablespoon canola oil

Direction:

1. Combine the ingredients in the bread pan by putting the wet ingredients first, followed by the dry ones.

2. Press the "Normal" or "Basic" mode and light the bread machine's crust colour setting.

3. After the cycles are completed, take out the bread from the machine.

4. Cooldown and then slice the bread.

Nutrition: Calories: 136 | Carbohydrates: 27g Fat: 2g | Protein: 3g

Vegan Cinnamon Raisin Bread

Preparation Time: 10 minutes

Cooking Time: 3 hours

Serving Size: 2 ounces (56.7g)

Ingredients:

- Two ¼ cups oat flour
- ¾ cup raisins
- ½ cup almond flour
- ¼ cup of coconut sugar
- 2 ½ teaspoons cinnamon
- One teaspoon baking powder
- ½ teaspoon baking soda
- ¼ teaspoon salt
- ¾ cup of water
- ½ cup of soy milk
- ¼ cup maple syrup
- Three tablespoons coconut oil
- One teaspoon vanilla extract

Direction:

1. Put all wet ingredients first into the bread pan, followed by the dry ingredients.
2. Set the bread machine to "Quick" or "Cake" mode.
3. Wait until the mixing and baking cycles are done.
4. Remove the pan from the machine.
5. Wait for another 10 minutes before transferring the bread to a wire rack.
6. After the bread has completely cooled down, slice it and serve.

Nutrition: Calories: 130 | Carbohydrates: 26g Fat: 2g | Protein: 3g

Beer Bread

Preparation Time: 10-15 minutes

Cooking Time: 2.5-3 hours

Serving Size: 2 ounces (56.7g)

Ingredients:

- 3 cups bread flour
- Two tablespoons sugar
- Two ¼ teaspoons yeast
- 1 ½ teaspoons salt
- 2/3 cup beer
- 1/3 cup water
- Two tablespoons vegetable oil

Direction:

1. Add all ingredients into a pan in this order: water, beer, oil, salt, sugar, flour, and yeast.
2. Start the bread machine with the "Basic" or "Normal" mode on and light to medium crust colour.
3. Let the machine complete all cycles.
4. Take out the pan from the machine.

5. Transfer the beer bread into a wire rack to cool it down for about an hour.

6. Cut into 12 slices, and serve.

Nutrition: Calories: 130 | Carbohydrates: 25g Fat: 1g | Protein: 4g

Onion and Mushroom Bread

Preparation Time: 10 minutes

Cooking Time: 1 hour

Serving Size: 2 ounces (56.7g)

Ingredients:

- 4 ounces mushrooms, chopped
- 4 cups bread flour
- Three tablespoons sugar
- Four teaspoons fast-acting yeast
- Four teaspoons dried onions, minced
- 1 ½ teaspoons salt
- ½ teaspoon garlic powder
- ¾ cup of water

Direction:

1. Pour the water first into the bread pan, and then add all of the dry ingredients.
2. Press the "Fast" cycle mode of the bread machine.
3. Wait until all cycles are completed.

4. Transfer the bread from the pan into a wire rack.

5. Wait for one hour before slicing the bread into 12 pieces.

6. Serving Size: 2 ounces per slice

Nutrition: Calories: 120 | Carbohydrates: 25g Fat: 0g | Protein: 5g

Low-Carb Multigrain Bread

Preparation Time: 15 minutes

Cooking Time: 1.5 hours

Serving Size: 1 ounce (28.3g)

Ingredients:

- ¾ cup whole-wheat flour
- ¼ cup cornmeal
- ¼ cup oatmeal
- Two tablespoons 7-grain cereals
- Two tablespoons baking powder
- One teaspoon salt
- ¼ teaspoon baking soda
- ¾ cup of water
- ¼ cup of vegetable oil
- ¼ cup of orange juice
- Three tablespoons aquafaba

Direction:

1. In the bread pan, add the wet ingredients first, then the dry ingredients.

2. Press the "Quick" or "Cake" mode of your bread machine.

3. Wait until all cycles are through.

4. Remove the bread pan from the machine.

5. Let the bread rest for 10 minutes in the pan before taking it out to cool down further.

6. Slice the bread after an hour has passed.

Nutrition: Calories: 60 | Carbohydrates: 9g Fat: 2g | Protein: 1g

Mashed Potato Bread

Preparation Time: 40 minutes

Cooking Time: 2.5-3 hours

Serving Size: 2 ounces (56.7g) per slice

Ingredients:

- 2 1/3 cups bread flour
- ½ cup mashed potatoes
- One tablespoon sugar
- 1 ½ teaspoons yeast
- ¾ teaspoon salt
- ¼ cup potato water
- One tablespoon ground flax seeds
- Four teaspoons oil

Direction:

1. Put the ingredients into the pan in this order: potato water, oil, flax seeds, mashed potatoes, sugar, salt, flour, and yeast.

2. Ready the bread machine by pressing the "Basic" or "Normal" mode with a medium crust colour setting.

3. Allow the bread machine to finish all cycles.

4. Remove the bread pan from the machine.

5. Carefully take the bread from the pan.

6. Put the bread on a wire rack, then cool down before slicing.

Nutrition: Calories: 140 Carbohydrates: 26 g

Healthy Celery Loaf

Preparation Time: 2 hours 40 minutes

Cooking Time: 50 minutes

Servings: 1 loaf

Ingredients:

- 1 can (10 ounces) cream of celery soup
- tablespoons low-fat milk, heated
- 1 tablespoon vegetable oil
- 1¼ teaspoons celery salt
- ¾ cup celery, fresh/sliced thin
- 1 tablespoon celery leaves, fresh, chopped
- 1 whole egg
- ¼ teaspoon sugar
- cups bread flour
- ¼ teaspoon ginger
- ½ cup quick-cooking oats
- tablespoons gluten
- teaspoons celery seeds
- 1 pack of active dry yeast

Directions:

1 Add all of the ingredients to your bread
   machine, carefully following the instructions
   of the manufacturer
2 Set the program of your bread machine to
   Basic/White Bread and set crust type to
   Medium
3 Press START
4 Wait until the cycle completes
5 Once the loaf is ready, take the bucket out
   and let the loaf cool for 5 minutes
6 Gently shake the bucket to remove the loaf
7 Transfer to a cooling rack, slice and serve
8 Enjoy!

Nutrition: Calories: 73 Cal Fat: 4 g
Carbohydrates: 8 g Protein: 3 g Fiber: 1 g

Broccoli and Cauliflower Bread

Preparation Time: 2 hours 20 minutes

Cooking Time: 50 minutes

Servings: 1 loaf

Ingredients:

- ¼ cup water
- tablespoons olive oil
- 1 egg white
- 1 teaspoon lemon juice
- 2/3 cup grated cheddar cheese
- tablespoons green onion
- ½ cup broccoli, chopped
- ½ cup cauliflower, chopped
- ½ teaspoon lemon pepper seasoning
- cups bread flour
- 1 teaspoon bread machine yeast

Directions:

1 Add all of the ingredients to your bread machine, carefully following the instructions of the manufacturer

2 Set the program of your bread machine to Basic/White Bread and set crust type to Medium

3 Press START

4 Wait until the cycle completes

5 Once the loaf is ready, take the bucket out and let the loaf cool for 5 minutes

6 Gently shake the bucket to remove the loaf

7 Transfer to a cooling rack, slice and serve

8 Enjoy!

Nutrition: Calories: 156 Cal Fat: 8 g Carbohydrates: 17 g Protein: 5 g Fiber: 2 g

Zucchini Herbed Bread

Preparation Time: 2 hours 20 minutes

Cooking Time: 50 minutes

Servings: 1 loaf

Ingredients:

- ½ cup water
- teaspoon honey
- 1 tablespoons oil
- ¾ cup zucchini, grated
- ¾ cup whole wheat flour
- cups bread flour
- 1 tablespoon fresh basil, chopped
- teaspoon sesame seeds
- 1 teaspoon salt
- 1½ teaspoon active dry yeast

Directions:

1 Add all of the ingredients to your bread machine, carefully following the instructions of the manufacturer

2 Set the program of your bread machine to Basic/White Bread and set crust type to Medium

3 Press START

4 Wait until the cycle completes

5 Once the loaf is ready, take the bucket out and let the loaf cool for 5 minutes

6 Gently shake the bucket to remove the loaf

7 Transfer to a cooling rack, slice and serve

8 Enjoy!

Nutrition: Calories: 153 Cal Fat: 1 g Carbohydrates: 28 g Protein: 5 g Fiber: 2 g

Potato Bread

Preparation Time: 3 hours

Cooking Time: 45 minutes

Servings: 2 loaves

Ingredients:

- 1 3/4 teaspoon active dry yeast
- tablespoon dry milk
- 1/4 cup instant potato flakes
- tablespoon sugar
- cups bread flour
- 1 1/4 teaspoon salt
- tablespoon butter
- 1 3/8 cups water

Directions:

1   Put all the liquid ingredients in the pan. Add all the dry ingredients, except the yeast. Form a shallow hole in the middle of the dry ingredients and place the yeast.

2 Secure the pan in the machine and close the lid. Choose the basic setting and your desired color of the crust. Press starts.

3 Allow the bread to cool before slicing.

Nutrition: Calories: 35calories; Total Carbohydrate: 19 g Total Fat: 0 g Protein: 4 g

Golden Potato Bread

Preparation Time: 2 hours 50 minutes

Cooking Time: 45 minutes

Servings: 2 loaves

Ingredients:

- teaspoon bread machine yeast
- cups bread flour
- 1 1/2 teaspoon salt
- tablespoon potato starch
- 1 tablespoon dried chives
- tablespoon dry skim milk powder
- 1 teaspoon sugar
- tablespoon unsalted butter, cubed
- 3/4 cup mashed potatoes
- 1 large egg, at room temperature
- 3/4 cup potato cooking water, with a temperature of 80 to 90 degrees F (26 to 32 degrees C)

Directions:

1 Prepare the mashed potatoes. Peel the potatoes and put them in a saucepan. Pour enough cold water to cover them. Turn the heat to high and bring to a boil. Turn the heat to low and continue cooking the potatoes until tender. Transfer the cooked potatoes to a bowl and mash. Cover the bowl until the potatoes are ready to use. Reserve cooking water and cook until it reaches the needed temperature.

2 Put the ingredients in the bread pan in this order: potato cooking water, egg, mashed potatoes, butter, sugar, milk, chives, potato starch, salt, flour, and yeast.

3 Place the pan in the machine and close the lid. Turn it on. Choose the sweet setting and your preferred crust color. Start the cooking process.

4 Gently unmold the baked bread and leave to cool on a wire rack.

5 Slice and serve.

Nutrition: Calories: 90calories; Total Carbohydrate: 15 g Total Fat: 2 g Protein: 4 g Protein: 4 g

Onion Potato Bread

Preparation Time: 1 hour 20 minutes

Cooking Time: 45 minutes

Servings: 2 loaves

Ingredients:

- tablespoon quick rise yeast
- cups bread flour
- 1 1/2 teaspoon seasoned salt
- tablespoon sugar
- 2/3 cup baked potatoes, mashed
- 1 1/2 cup onions, minced
- large eggs
- tablespoon oil
- 3/4 cup hot water, with the temperature of 115 to 125 degrees F (46 to 51 degrees C)

Directions:

1 Put the liquid ingredients in the pan. Add the dry ingredients, except the yeast. Form a shallow well in the middle using your hand and put the yeast.

2   Place the pan in the machine, close the lid and turn it on. Select the express bake 80 setting and start the machine.

3   Once the bread is cooked, leave on a wire rack for 20 minutes or until cooled.

Nutrition: Calories: 160calories; Total Carbohydrate: 44 g Total Fat: 2 g Protein: 6 g

Spinach Bread

Preparation Time: 2 hours 20 minutes

Cooking Time: 40 minutes

Servings: 1 loaf

Ingredients:

- 1 cup water
- 1 tablespoon vegetable oil
- 1/2 cup frozen chopped spinach, thawed and drained
- cups all-purpose flour
- 1/2 cup shredded Cheddar cheese
- 1 teaspoon salt
- 1 tablespoon white sugar
- 1/2 teaspoon ground black pepper
- 1/2 teaspoons active dry yeast

Directions:

1 In the pan of bread machine, put all ingredients according to the suggested order of manufacture. Set white bread cycle.

Nutrition: Calories: 121 calories; Total Carbohydrate: 20.5 g Cholesterol: 4 mg Total Fat: 2.5 g Protein: 4 g Sodium: 184 mg

Curd Bread

Preparation Time: 4 hours

Cooking Time: 15 minutes

Servings: 12

Ingredients:

- ¾ cup lukewarm water
- 2/3 cups wheat bread machine flour
- ¾ cup cottage cheese
- Tablespoon softened butter
- Tablespoon white sugar
- 1½ teaspoon sea salt
- 1½ Tablespoon sesame seeds
- Tablespoon dried onions
- 1¼ teaspoon bread machine yeast

Directions:

2 Place all the dry and liquid ingredients in the pan and follow the instructions for your bread machine.

3 Pay particular attention to measuring the ingredients. Use a measuring cup,

measuring spoon, and kitchen scales to do so.

4 Set the baking program to BASIC and the crust type to MEDIUM.

5 If the dough is too dense or too wet, adjust the amount of flour and liquid in the recipe.

6 When the program has ended, take the pan out of the bread machine and let cool for 5 minutes.

7 Shake the loaf out of the pan. If necessary, use a spatula.

8 Wrap the bread with a kitchen towel and set it aside for an hour. Otherwise, you can cool it on a wire rack.

Nutrition: Calories: 277 calories; Total Carbohydrate: 48.4 g Cholesterol: 9 g Total Fat: 4.7g Protein: 9.4 g Sodium: 547 mg Sugar: 3.3 g

Curvy Carrot Bread

Preparation Time: 2 hours

Cooking Time: 15 minutes

Servings: 12

Ingredients:

- ¾ cup milk, lukewarm
- tablespoons butter, melted at room temperature
- 1 tablespoon honey
- ¾ teaspoon ground nutmeg
- ½ teaspoon salt
- 1 ½ cups shredded carrot
- cups white bread flour
- ¼ teaspoons bread machine or active dry yeast

Directions:

1 Take 1 ½ pound size loaf pan and first add the liquid ingredients and then add the dry ingredients.

2 Place the loaf pan in the machine and close its top lid.

3 Plug the bread machine into power socket. For selecting a bread cycle, press "Quick Bread/Rapid Bread" and for selecting a crust type, press "Light" or "Medium".

4 Start the machine and it will start preparing the bread.

5 After the bread loaf is completed, open the lid and take out the loaf pan.

6 Allow the pan to cool down for 10-15 minutes on a wire rack. Gently shake the pan and remove the bread loaf.

7 Make slices and serve.

Nutrition: Calories: 142 calories; Total Carbohydrate: 32.2 g Cholesterol: 0 g Total Fat: 0.8 g Protein: 2.33 g

Potato Rosemary Bread

Preparation Time: 3 hours

Cooking Time: 30 minutes

Servings: 20

Ingredients:

- cups bread flour, sifted
- 1 tablespoon white sugar
- 1 tablespoon sunflower oil
- 1½ teaspoons salt
- 1½ cups lukewarm water
- 1 teaspoon active dry yeast
- 1 cup potatoes, mashed
- teaspoons crushed rosemary

Directions:

1 Prepare all of the ingredients for your bread and measuring means (a cup, a spoon, kitchen scales).

2 Carefully measure the ingredients into the pan, except the potato and rosemary.

3 Place all of the ingredients into the bread
   bucket in the right order, following the
   manual for your bread machine.

4 Close the cover.

5 Select the program of your bread machine to
   BREAD with FILLINGS and choose the crust
   color to MEDIUM.

6 Press START.

7 After the signal, put the mashed potato and
   rosemary to the dough.

8 Wait until the program completes.

9 When done, take the bucket out and let it
   cool for 5-10 minutes.

10 Shake the loaf from the pan and let cool for
   30 minutes on a cooling rack.

11 Slice, serve and enjoy the taste of fragrant
   homemade bread.

Nutrition: Calories: 106 calories; Total
Carbohydrate: 21 g Total Fat: 1 g Protein: 2.9 g
Sodium: 641 mg Fiber: 1 g Sugar: 0.8 g

Beetroot Prune Bread

Preparation Time: 3 hours

Cooking Time: 30 minutes

Servings: 20

Ingredients:

- 1½ cups lukewarm beet broth
- 5¼ cups all-purpose flour
- 1 cup beet puree
- 1 cup prunes, chopped
- tablespoons extra virgin olive oil
- tablespoons dry cream
- 1 tablespoon brown sugar
- teaspoons active dry yeast
- 1 tablespoon whole milk
- teaspoons sea salt

Directions:

1 Prepare all of the ingredients for your bread and measuring means (a cup, a spoon, kitchen scales).

2 Carefully measure the ingredients into the pan, except the prunes.

3 Place all of the ingredients into the bread bucket in the right order, following the manual for your bread machine.

4 Close the cover.

5 Select the program of your bread machine to BASIC and choose the crust color to MEDIUM.

6 Press START.

7 After the signal, put the prunes to the dough.

8 Wait until the program completes.

9 When done, take the bucket out and let it cool for 5-10 minutes.

10 Shake the loaf from the pan and let cool for 30 minutes on a cooling rack.

11 Slice, serve and enjoy the taste of fragrant homemade bread.

Nutrition: Calories: 443 calories; Total Carbohydrate: 81.1 g Total Fat: 8.2 g Protein: 9.9 g Sodium: 604 mg Fiber: 4.4 g Sugar: 11.7 g

SAUCES, DRESSINGS, AND DIPS

Satay Sauce

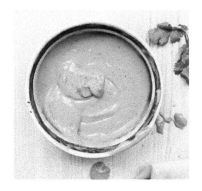

Preparation Time: 5 minutes

Cooking Time: 8 minutes

Servings: 2

Ingredients:

- ½ yellow onion, diced
- 3 garlic cloves, minced
- 1 fresh red chile, thinly sliced (optional)
- 1-inch (2.5-cm) piece fresh ginger, peeled and minced

- ¼ cup smooth peanut butter
- 2 tablespoons coconut aminos
- 1 (13.5-ounce / 383-g) can unsweetened coconut milk
- ¼ teaspoon freshly ground black pepper
- ¼ teaspoon salt (optional)

Directions:

1. Heat a large nonstick skillet over medium-high heat until hot.
2. Add the onion, garlic cloves, chile (if desired), and ginger to the skillet, and sauté for 2 minutes.
3. Pour in the peanut butter and coconut aminos and stir well. Add the coconut milk, black pepper, and salt (if desired) and continue whisking, or until the sauce is just beginning to bubble and thicken.
4. Remove the sauce from the heat to a bowl. Taste and adjust the seasoning if necessary.

Nutrition: Calories: 322 Fat: 28.8g Carbs: 9.4g Protein: 6.3g Fiber: 1.8g

Tahini BBQ Sauce

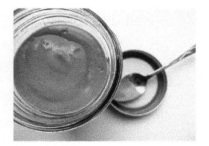

Preparation Time: 10 minutes

Cooking Time: 0 minutes

Servings: 4

Ingredients:

- ½ cup water
- ¼ cup red miso
- 3 cloves garlic, minced
- 1-inch (2.5 cm) piece ginger, peeled and minced
- 2 tablespoons rice vinegar
- 2 tablespoons tahini
- 2 tablespoons chili paste or chili sauce
- 1 tablespoon date sugar
- ½ teaspoon crushed red pepper (optional)

Directions:

1. Place all the ingredients in a food processor, and purée until thoroughly mixed and smooth. You

can thin the sauce out by stirring in ½ cup of water, or keep it thick.

2. Transfer to the refrigerator to chill until ready to serve.

Nutrition: Calories: 206 Fat: 10.2g Carbs: 21.3g Protein: 7.2g Fiber: 4.4g

Tamari Vinegar Sauce

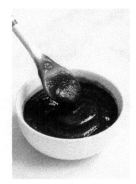

Preparation Time: 10 minutes

Cooking Time: 0 minutes

Servings: 1

Ingredients:

- ¼ cup tamari
- ½ cup nutritional yeast
- 2 tablespoons balsamic vinegar
- 2 tablespoons apple cider vinegar
- 2 tablespoons Worcestershire sauce
- 2 teaspoons Dijon mustard
- 1 tablespoon plus 1 teaspoon maple syrup
- ½ teaspoon ground turmeric
- ¼ teaspoon black pepper

Directions:

1. Place all the ingredients in an airtight container, and whisk until everything is well incorporated. Store in the refrigerator for up to 3 weeks.

Nutrition: Calories: 216 Fat: 9.9g Carbs: 18.0g Protein: 13.7g Fiber: 7.7g

Sweet and Tangy Ketchup

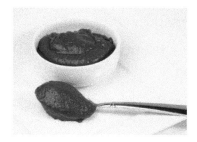

Preparation Time: 5 minutes

Cooking Time: 15 minutes

Servings: 2

Ingredients:

- 1 cup water
- ¼ cup maple syrup
- 1 cup tomato paste
- 3 tablespoons apple cider vinegar
- 1 teaspoon onion powder
- 1 teaspoon garlic powder

Directions:

1. Add the water to a medium saucepan and bring to a rolling boil over high heat.
2. Reduce the heat to low, stir in the maple syrup, tomato paste, vinegar, onion powder, and garlic powder. Cover and bring to a gently simmer for

about 10 minutes, stirring frequently, or until the sauce begins to thicken and bubble.

3. Let the sauce rest for 30 minutes until cooled completely. Transfer to an airtight container and refrigerate for up to 1 month.

Nutrition: Calories: 46 Fat: 5.2g Carbs: 1.0g Protein: 1.1g Fiber: 1.0g

Homemade Tzatziki Sauce

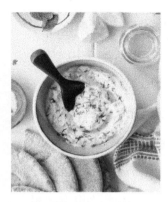

Preparation Time: 20 minutes

Cooking Time: 0 minutes

Servings: 1

Ingredients:

- 2 ounces (57 g) raw, unsalted cashews (about ½ cup)
- 2 tablespoons lemon juice
- 1/3 cup water
- 1 small clove garlic
- 1 cup chopped cucumber, peeled
- 2 tablespoons fresh dill

Directions:

1. In a blender, add the cashews, lemon juice, water, and garlic. Keep it aside for at least 15 minutes to soften the cashews.

2. Blend the ingredients until smooth. Stir in the chopped cucumber and dill, and continue to blend until it reaches your desired consistency. It doesn't need to be totally smooth. Feel free to add more water if you like a thinner consistency.

3. Transfer to an airtight container and chill for at least 30 minutes for best flavors.

4. Bring the sauce to room temperature and shake well before serving.

Nutrition: Calories: 208 Fat: 13.5g Carbs: 15.0 g Protein: 6.7g Fiber: 2.8g

Tangy Cashew Mustard Dressing

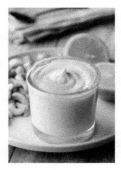

Preparation Time: 20 minutes

Cooking Time: 0 minutes

Servings: 1

Ingredients:

- 2 ounces (57 g) raw, unsalted cashews (about ½ cup)
- ½ cup water
- 3 tablespoons lemon juice
- 2 teaspoons apple cider vinegar
- 2 tablespoons Dijon mustard
- 1 medium clove garlic

Directions:

1. Put all the ingredients in a food processor and keep it aside for at least 15 minutes.

---

2. Purée until the ingredients are combined to a smooth and creamy mixture. Thin the dressing with a little extra water as needed to achieve your preferred consistency.
3. Store in an airtight container in the refrigerator for up to 5 days.

Nutrition: Calories: 187 Fat: 13.0g Carbs: 11.5g Protein: 5.9g Fiber: 1.7g

Avocado-dill Dressing

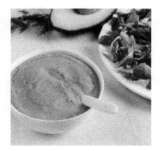

Preparation Time: 20 minutes

Cooking Time: 0 minutes

Servings: 1

Ingredients:

- 2 ounces (57 g) raw, unsalted cashews (about ½ cup)
- ½ cup water
- 3 tablespoons lemon juice
- ½ medium, ripe avocado, chopped
- 1 medium clove garlic
- 2 tablespoons chopped fresh dill
- 2 green onions, white and green parts, chopped

Directions:

1. Put the cashews, water, lemon juice, avocado, and garlic into a blender. Keep it aside for at least 15 minutes to soften the cashews.
2. Blend until everything is fully mixed. Fold in the dill and green onions, and blend briefly to retain some texture.
3. Store in an airtight container in the fridge for up to 3 days and stir well before serving.

Nutrition: Calories: 312 Fat: 21.1g Carbs: 22.6g Protein: 8.0g Fiber: 7.1g

Easy Lemon Tahini Dressing

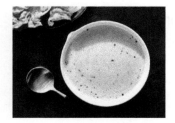

Preparation Time: 5 minutes

Cooking Time: 0 minutes

Servings: 1

Ingredients:

- ½ cup tahini
- ¼ cup fresh lemon juice (about 2 lemons)
- 1 teaspoon maple syrup
- 1 small garlic clove, chopped
- 1/8 teaspoon black pepper
- ¼ teaspoon salt (optional)
- ¼ to ½ cup water

Directions:

1. Process the tahini, lemon juice, maple syrup, garlic, black pepper, and salt (if desired) in a blender (high-speed blenders work best for this).

Gradually add the water until the mixture is completely smooth.

2. Store in an airtight container in the fridge for up to 5 days.

Nutrition: Calories: 128 Fat: 9.6g Carbs: 6.8g Protein: 3.6g Fiber: 1.9g

Sweet Mango and Orange Dressing

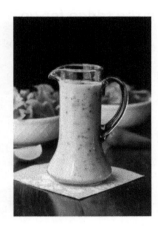

Preparation Time: 5 minutes

Cooking Time: 0 minutes

Servings: 1

Ingredients:

- 1 cup (165 g) diced mango, thawed if frozen
- ½ cup orange juice
- 2 tablespoons rice vinegar
- 2 tablespoons fresh lime juice
- ¼ teaspoon salt (optional)
- 1 teaspoon date sugar (optional)
- 2 tablespoons chopped cilantro

Directions:

1. Pulse all the ingredients except for the cilantro in a food processor until it reaches the consistency you like. Add the cilantro and whisk well.
2. Store in an airtight container in the fridge for up to 2 days.

Nutrition: Calories: 32 Fat: 0.1g Carbs: 7.4g Protein: 0.3g Fiber: 0.5g

SALADS RECIPES

Cashew Siam Salad

Preparation Time: 10 minutes

Cooking Time: 3 minutes

Servings: 4

Ingredients:

Salad:

- 4 cups baby spinach, rinsed, drained
- ½ cup pickled red cabbage

Dressing:

- 1-inch piece ginger, finely chopped
- 1 tsp. chili garlic paste
- 1 tbsp. soy sauce
- ½ tbsp. rice vinegar
- 1 tbsp. sesame oil
- 3 tbsp. avocado oil

Toppings:

- ½ cup raw cashews, unsalted
- ¼ cup fresh cilantro, chopped

Directions:

1. Put the spinach and red cabbage in a large bowl. Toss to combine and set the salad aside.

2. Toast the cashews in a frying pan over medium-high heat, stirring occasionally until the cashews are golden brown. This should take about 3 minutes. Turn off the heat and set the frying pan aside.

3. Mix all the dressing ingredients in medium-sized bowl and use a spoon to mix them into a smooth dressing.

4. Pour the dressing over the spinach salad and top with the toasted cashews.

5. Toss the salad to combine all ingredients and transfer the large bowl to the fridge. Allow the salad to chill for up to one hour – doing so will guarantee a better flavor. Alternatively, the salad can be served right away, topped with the optional cilantro. Enjoy!

Nutrition: Calories 160 Total Fat 12.9g Saturated Fat 2.4g Cholesterol 0mg Sodium 265mg Total Carbohydrate 9.1g Dietary Fiber 2.1g Total Sugars

1.4g Protein 4.1g Vitamin D 0mcg Calcium 45mg
Iron 2mg Potassium 344mg

Cucumber Edamame Salad

Preparation Time: 5 minutes

Cooking Time: 8 minutes

Servings: 2

Ingredients:

- 3 tbsp. avocado oil
- 1 cup cucumber, sliced into thin rounds
- ½ cup fresh sugar snap peas, sliced or whole
- ½ cup fresh edamame
- ¼ cup radish, sliced
- 1 large Hass avocado, peeled, pitted, sliced
- 1 nori sheet, crumbled
- 2 tsp. roasted sesame seeds
- 1 tsp. salt

Directions:

1. Bring a medium-sized pot filled half way with water to a boil over medium-high heat.
2. Add the sugar snaps and cook them for about 2 minutes.

3. Take the pot off the heat, drain the excess water, transfer the sugar snaps to a medium-sized bowl and set aside for now.

4. Fill the pot with water again, add the teaspoon of salt and bring to a boil over medium-high heat.

5. Add the edamame to the pot and let them cook for about 6 minutes.

6. Take the pot off the heat, drain the excess water, transfer the soybeans to the bowl with sugar snaps and let them cool down for about 5 minutes.

7. Combine all ingredients, except the nori crumbs and roasted sesame seeds, in a medium-sized bowl.

8. Carefully stir, using a spoon, until all ingredients are evenly coated in oil.

9. Top the salad with the nori crumbs and roasted sesame seeds.

10. Transfer the bowl to the fridge and allow the salad to cool for at least 30 minutes.

11. Serve chilled and enjoy!

Nutrition: Calories 182 Total Fat 10.9g Saturated Fat 1.3g Cholesterol 0mg Sodium 1182mg Total Carbohydrate 14.2g Dietary Fiber 5.4g Total Sugars 1.9g Protein 10.7g Vitamin D 0mcg, Calcium 181mg Iron 4mg Potassium 619mg

Spinach and Mashed Tofu Salad

Preparation Time: 20 minutes

Cooking Time: 0 minutes

Servings: 4

Ingredients:

- 2 8-oz. blocks firm tofu, drained
- 4 cups baby spinach leaves
- 4 tbsp. cashew butter
- 1½ tbsp. soy sauce
- 1tbsp ginger, chopped
- 1 tsp. red miso paste
- 2 tbsp. sesame seeds
- 1 tsp. organic orange zest
- 1 tsp. nori flakes
- 2 tbsp. water

Directions:

1. Use paper towels to absorb any excess water left in the tofu before crumbling both blocks into small pieces.
2. In a large bowl, combine the mashed tofu with the spinach leaves.

3. Mix the remaining ingredients in another small bowl and, if desired, add the optional water for a more smooth dressing.

4. Pour this dressing over the mashed tofu and spinach leaves.

5. Transfer the bowl to the fridge and allow the salad to chill for up to one hour. Doing so will guarantee a better flavor. Or, the salad can be served right away. Enjoy!

Nutrition: Calories 623 Total Fat 30.5g Saturated Fat 5.8g Cholesterol 0mg Sodium 2810mg Total Carbohydrate 48g Dietary Fiber 5.9g Total Sugars 3g Protein 48.4g Vitamin D 0mcg Calcium 797mg Iron 22mg Potassium 2007mg

Super Summer Salad

Preparation Time: 10 minutes

Cooking Time: 0 minutes

Servings: 2

Ingredients:

Dressing:

- 1 tbsp. olive oil
- ¼ cup chopped basil
- 1 tsp. lemon juice
- ¼ tsp Salt
- 1 medium avocado, halved, diced
- ¼ cup water

Salad:

- ¼ cup dry chickpeas
- ¼ cup dry red kidney beans
- 4 cups raw kale, shredded
- 2 cups Brussel sprouts, shredded
- 2 radishes, thinly sliced
- 1 tbsp. walnuts, chopped
- 1 tsp. flax seeds
- Salt and pepper to taste

Directions:

1. Prepare the chickpeas and kidney beans according to the method.
2. Soak the flax seeds according the method, and then drain excess water.
3. Prepare the dressing by adding the olive oil, basil, lemon juice, salt, and half of the avocado to a food processor or blender, and pulse on low speed.
4. Keep adding small amounts of water until the dressing is creamy and smooth.
5. Transfer the dressing to a small bowl and set it aside.
6. Combine the kale, Brussel sprouts, cooked chickpeas, kidney beans, radishes, walnuts, and remaining avocado in a large bowl and mix thoroughly.
7. Store the mixture, or, serve with the dressing and flax seeds, and enjoy!

Nutrition: Calories 266 Total Fat 26.6g Saturated Fat 5.1g Cholesterol 0mg Sodium 298mg Total Carbohydrate 8.8g Dietary Fiber 6.8g Total Sugars

0.6g Protein 2g Vitamin D 0mcg Calcium 19mg
Iron 1mg Potassium 500mg

Roasted Almond Protein Salad

Preparation Time: 30 minutes

Cooking Time: 0 minutes

Servings: 4

Ingredients:

- ½ cup dry quinoa
- ½ cup dry navy beans
- ½ cup dry chickpeas
- ½ cup raw whole almonds
- 1 tsp. extra virgin olive oil
- ½ tsp. salt
- ½ tsp. paprika
- ½ tsp. cayenne
- Dash of chili powder
- 4 cups spinach, fresh or frozen
- ¼ cup purple onion, chopped

Directions:

1. Prepare the quinoa according to the recipe. Store in the fridge for now.
2. Prepare the beans according to the method. Store in the fridge for now.

3. Toss the almonds, olive oil, salt, and spices in a large bowl, and stir until the ingredients are evenly coated.
4. Put a skillet over medium-high heat, and transfer the almond mixture to the heated skillet.
5. Roast while stirring until the almonds are browned, around 5 minutes. You may hear the ingredients pop and crackle in the pan as they warm up. Stir frequently to prevent burning.
6. Turn off the heat and toss the cooked and chilled quinoa and beans, onions, and spinach or mixed greens in the skillet. Stir well before transferring the roasted almond salad to a bowl.
7. Enjoy the salad with a dressing of choice, or, store for later!

Nutrition: Calories 347 Total Fat 10.5g Saturated Fat 1g Cholesterol 0mg Sodium 324mg Total Carbohydrate 49.2g Dietary Fiber 14.7g Total Sugars 4.7g Protein 17.2g Vitamin D 0mcg Calcium 139mg Iron 5mg Potassium 924mg

Lentil, Lemon & Mushroom Salad

Preparation Time: 10 minutes

Cooking Time: 0 minutes

Servings: 2

Ingredients:

- ½ cup dry lentils of choice
- 2 cups vegetable broth
- 3 cups mushrooms, thickly sliced
- 1 cup sweet or purple onion, chopped
- 4 tsp. extra virgin olive oil
- 2 tbsp. garlic powder
- ¼ tsp. chili flakes
- 1 tbsp. lemon juice
- 2 tbsp. cilantro, chopped
- ½ cup arugula
- ¼ tsp Salt
- ¼ tsp pepper

Directions:

1. Sprout the lentils according the method. (Don't cook them).

2. Place the vegetable stock in a deep saucepan and bring it to a boil.
3. Add the lentils to the boiling broth, cover the pan, and cook for about 5 minutes over low heat until the lentils are a bit tender.
4. Remove the pan from heat and drain the excess water.
5. Put a frying pan over high heat and add 2 tablespoons of olive oil.
6. Add the onions, garlic, and chili flakes, and cook until the onions are almost translucent, around 5 to 10 minutes while stirring.
7. Add the mushrooms to the frying pan and mix in thoroughly. Continue cooking until the onions are completely translucent and the mushrooms have softened; remove the pan from the heat.
8. Mix the lentils, onions, mushrooms, and garlic in a large bowl.
9. Add the lemon juice and the remaining olive oil. Toss or stir to combine everything thoroughly.
10. Serve the mushroom/onion mixture over some arugala in bowl, adding salt and pepper to taste, or, store and enjoy later!

Nutrition: Calories 365 Total Fat 11.7g Saturated Fat 1.9g Cholesterol 0mg Sodium 1071mg Total Carbohydrate 45.2g Dietary Fiber 18g Total Sugars 8.2g Protein 22.8g Vitamin D 378mcg Calcium 67mg Iron 8mg Potassium 1212mg

Sweet Potato & Black Bean Protein Salad

Preparation Time: 15 minutes

Cooking Time: 0 minutes

Servings: 2

Ingredients:

- 1 cup dry black beans
- 4 cups of spinach
- 1 medium sweet potato
- 1 cup purple onion, chopped
- 2 tbsp. olive oil
- 2 tbsp. lime juice
- 1 tbsp. minced garlic
- ½ tbsp. chili powder
- ¼ tsp. cayenne
- ¼ cup parsley
- ¼ tsp Salt
- ¼ tsp pepper

Directions:

1. Prepare the black beans according to the method.

2. Preheat the oven to 400°F.

3. Cut the sweet potato into ¼-inch cubes and put these in a medium-sized bowl. Add the onions, 1 tablespoon of olive oil, and salt to taste.

4. Toss the ingredients until the sweet potatoes and onions are completely coated.

5. Transfer the ingredients to a baking sheet lined with parchment paper and spread them out in a single layer.

6. Put the baking sheet in the oven and roast until the sweet potatoes are starting to turn brown and crispy, around 40 minutes.

7. Meanwhile, combine the remaining olive oil, lime juice, garlic, chili powder, and cayenne thoroughly in a large bowl, until no lumps remain.

8. Remove the sweet potatoes and onions from the oven and transfer them to the large bowl.

9. Add the cooked black beans, parsley, and a pinch of salt.

10. Toss everything until well combined.

11. Then mix in the spinach, and serve in desired portions with additional salt and pepper.

12.Store or enjoy!

Nutrition: Calories 558 Total Fat 16.2g Saturated Fat 2.5g Cholesterol 0mg Sodium 390mg Total Carbohydrate 84g Dietary Fiber 20.4g Total Sugars 8.9g Protein 25.3g Vitamin D 0mcg Calcium 220mg Iron 10mg Potassium 2243mg

Lentil Radish Salad

Preparation Time: 15 minutes

Cooking Time: 0 minutes

Servings: 3

Ingredients:

Dressing:

- 1 tbsp. extra virgin olive oil
- 1 tbsp. lemon juice
- 1 tbsp. maple syrup
- 1 tbsp. water
- ½ tbsp. sesame oil
- 1 tbsp. miso paste, yellow or white
- ¼ tsp. salt
- ¼ tsp Pepper

Salad:

- ½ cup dry chickpeas
- ¼ cup dry green or brown lentils
- 1 14-oz. pack of silken tofu
- 5 cups mixed greens, fresh or frozen
- 2 radishes, thinly sliced
- ½ cup cherry tomatoes, halved

- ¼ cup roasted sesame seeds

Directions:

1. Prepare the chickpeas according to the method.

2. Prepare the lentils according to the method.

3. Put all the ingredients for the dressing in a blender or food processor. Mix on low until smooth, while adding water until it reaches the desired consistency.

4. Add salt, pepper (to taste), and optionally more water to the dressing; set aside.

5. Cut the tofu into bite-sized cubes.

6. Combine the mixed greens, tofu, lentils, chickpeas, radishes, and tomatoes in a large bowl.

7. Add the dressing and mix everything until it is coated evenly.

8. Top with the optional roasted sesame seeds, if desired.

9. Refrigerate before serving and enjoy, or, store for later!

Nutrition: Calories 621 Total Fat 19.6g Saturated Fat 2.8g Cholesterol 0mg Sodium 996mg Total

Carbohydrate 82.7g Dietary Fiber 26.1g Total Sugars 20.7g Protein 31.3g Vitamin D 0mcg Calcium 289mg Iron 9mg Potassium 1370mg

Southwest Style Salad

Preparation Time: 10 minutes

Cooking Time: 0 minutes

Servings: 3

Ingredients:

- ½ cup dry black beans
- ½ cup dry chickpeas
- 1/3 cup purple onion, diced
- 1 red bell pepper, pitted, sliced
- 4 cups mixed greens, fresh or frozen, chopped
- 1 cup cherry tomatoes, halved or quartered
- 1 medium avocado, peeled, pitted, and cubed
- 1 cup sweet kernel corn, canned, drained
- ½ tsp. chili powder
- ¼ tsp. cumin
- ¼ tsp Salt
- ¼ tsp pepper
- 2 tsp. olive oil
- 1 tbsp. vinegar

Directions:

1. Prepare the black beans and chickpeas according to the method.
2. Put all of the ingredients into a large bowl.
3. Toss the mix of veggies and spices until combined thoroughly.
4. Store, or serve chilled with some olive oil and vinegar on top!

Nutrition: Calories 635 Total Fat 19.9g Saturated Fat 3.6g Cholesterol 0mg Sodium 302mg Total Carbohydrate 95.4g Dietary Fiber 28.1g Total Sugars 18.8g Protein 24.3g Vitamin D 0mcg Calcium 160mg Iron 7mg Potassium 1759mg

Shaved Brussel Sprout Salad

Preparation Time: 25 minutes

Cooking Time: 0 minutes

Servings: 4

Ingredients:

Dressing:

- 1 tbsp. brown mustard
- 1 tbsp. maple syrup
- 2 tbsp. apple cider vinegar
- 2 tbsp. extra virgin olive oil
- ½ tbsp. garlic minced

Salad:

- ½ cup dry red kidney beans
- ¼ cup dry chickpeas
- 2 cups Brussel sprouts
- 1 cup purple onion
- 1 small sour apple
- ½ cup slivered almonds, crushed
- ½ cup walnuts, crushed
- ½ cup cranberries, dried
- ¼ tsp Salt

- ¼ tsp pepper

Directions:

1. Prepare the beans according to the method.
2. Combine all dressing ingredients in a bowl and stir well until combined.
3. Refrigerate the dressing for up to one hour before serving.
4. Using a grater, mandolin, or knife to thinly slice each Brussel sprout. Repeat this with the apple and onion.
5. Take a large bowl to mix the chickpeas, beans, sprouts, apples, onions, cranberries, and nuts.
6. Drizzle the cold dressing over the salad to coat.
7. Serve with salt and pepper to taste, or, store for later!

Nutrition: Calories 432 Total Fat 23.5g Saturated Fat 2.2g Cholesterol 0mg Sodium 197mg Total Carbohydrate 45.3g Dietary Fiber 12.4g Total Sugars 14g Protein 15.9g Vitamin D 0mcg Calcium 104mg Iron 4mg Potassium 908mg

Colorful Protein Power Salad

Preparation Time: 20 minutes

Cooking Time: 0 minutes

Servings: 2

Ingredients:

- ½ cup dry quinoa
- 2 cups dry navy beans
- 1 green onion, chopped
- 2 tsp. garlic, minced
- 3 cups green or purple cabbage, chopped
- 4 cups kale, fresh or frozen, chopped
- 1 cup shredded carrot, chopped
- 2 tbsp. extra virgin olive oil
- 1 tsp. lemon juice
- ¼ tsp Salt
- ¼ tsp pepper

Directions:

1. Prepare the quinoa according to the recipe.
2. Prepare the beans according to the method.
3. Heat up 1 tablespoon of the olive oil in a frying pan over medium heat.

4. Add the chopped green onion, garlic, and cabbage, and sauté for 2-3 minutes.

5. Add the kale, the remaining 1 tablespoon of olive oil, and salt. Lower the heat and cover until the greens have wilted, around 5 minutes. Remove the pan from the stove and set aside.

6. Take a large bowl and mix the remaining ingredients with the kale and cabbage mixture once it has cooled down. Add more salt and pepper to taste.

7. Mix until everything is distributed evenly.

8. Serve topped with a dressing, or, store for later!

Nutrition: Calories 1100 Total Fat 19.9g Saturated Fat 2.7g Cholesterol 0mg Sodium 420mg Total Carbohydrate 180.8g Dietary Fiber 60.1g Total Sugars 14.4g Protein 58.6g Vitamin D 0mcg Calcium 578mg Iron 16mg Potassium 3755mg

Edamame & Ginger Citrus Salad

Preparation Time: 15 minutes

Cooking Time: 0 minutes

Servings: 3

Ingredients:

Dressing:

- ¼ cup orange juice
- 1 tsp. lime juice
- ½ tbsp. maple syrup
- ½ tsp. ginger, finely minced
- ½ tbsp. sesame oil

Salad:

- ½ cup dry green lentils
- 2 cups carrots, shredded
- 4 cups kale, fresh or frozen, chopped
- 1 cup edamame, shelled
- 1 tablespoon roasted sesame seeds
- 2 tsp. mint, chopped
- Salt and pepper to taste
- 1 small avocado, peeled, pitted, diced

Directions:

1. Prepare the lentils according to the method.

2. Combine the orange and lime juices, maple syrup, and ginger in a small bowl. Mix with a whisk while slowly adding the sesame oil.

3. Add the cooked lentils, carrots, kale, edamame, sesame seeds, and mint to a large bowl.

4. Add the dressing and stir well until all the ingredients are coated evenly.

5. Store or serve topped with avocado and an additional sprinkle of mint.

Nutrition: Calories 507 Total Fat 23.1g Saturated Fat 4g Cholesterol 0mg Sodium 303mg Total Carbohydrate 56.8g Dietary Fiber 21.6g Total Sugars 8.4g Protein 24.6g Vitamin D 0mcg Calcium 374mg Iron 8mg Potassium 1911mg

Taco Tempeh Salad

Preparation Time: 25 minutes

Cooking Time: 0 minutes

Servings: 3

Ingredients:

- 1 cup dry black beans
- 1 8-oz. package tempeh
- 1 tbsp. lime or lemon juice
- 2 tbsp. extra virgin olive oil
- 1 tsp. maple syrup
- ½ tsp. chili powder
- ¼ tsp. cumin
- ¼ tsp. paprika
- 1 large bunch of kale, fresh or frozen, chopped
- 1 large avocado, peeled, pitted, diced
- ½ cup salsa
- ¼ tsp Salt
- ¼ tsp pepper

Directions:

1. Prepare the beans according to the method.

2. Cut the tempeh into ¼-inch cubes, place in a bowl, and then add the lime or lemon juice, 1 tablespoon of olive oil, maple syrup, chili powder, cumin, and paprika.
3. Stir well and let the tempeh marinate in the fridge for at least 1 hour, up to 12 hours.
4. Heat the remaining 1 tablespoon of olive oil in a frying pan over medium heat.
5. Add the marinated tempeh mixture and cook until brown and crispy on both sides, around 10 minutes.
6. Put the chopped kale in a bowl with the cooked beans and prepared tempeh.
7. Store, or serve the salad immediately, topped with salsa, avocado, and salt and pepper to taste.

Nutrition: Calories 627 Total Fat 31.7g Saturated Fat 6.1g Cholesterol 0mg Sodium 493mg Total Carbohydrate 62.7g Dietary Fiber 16g Total Sugars 4.5g Protein 31.4g Vitamin D 0mcg Calcium 249mg Iron 7mg Potassium 1972mg

Lebanese Potato Salad

Preparation Time: 5 minutes

Cooking Time: 10 minutes

Servings: 4

Ingredients:

- 1-pound Russet potatoes
- 1 ½ tablespoons extra virgin olive oil
- 2 scallions, thinly sliced
- Freshly ground pepper to taste
- 2 tablespoons lemon juice
- ¼ teaspoon salt or to taste
- 2 tablespoons fresh mint leaves, chopped

Directions:

1. Place a saucepan half filled with water over medium heat. Add salt and potatoes and cook for 10 minutes until tender. Drain the potatoes and place in a bowl of cold water. When cool enough to handle, peel and cube the potatoes. Place in a bowl.

To make dressing:

2. Add oil, lemon juice, salt and pepper in a bowl and whisk well. Drizzle dressing over the potatoes. Toss well.
3. Add scallions and mint and toss well.
4. Divide into 4 plates and serve.

Nutrition: Calories 129 Total Fat 5.5g Saturated Fat 0.9g Cholesterol 0mg Sodium 158mg Total Carbohydrate 18.8g Dietary Fiber 3.2g Total Sugars 1.6g Protein 2.2g Vitamin D 0mcg Calcium 22mg Iron 1mg Potassium 505mg

Chickpea and Spinach Salad

Preparation Time: 5 minutes

Cooking Time: 0 minutes

Servings: 4

Ingredients:

- 2 cans (14.5 ounces each) chickpeas, drained, rinsed
- 7 ounces vegan feta cheese, crumbled or chopped
- 1 tablespoon lemon juice
- 1/3 -½ cup olive oil
- ½ teaspoon salt or to taste
- 4-6 cups spinach, torn
- ½ cup raisins
- 2 tablespoons honey
- 1-2 teaspoons ground cumin
- 1 teaspoon chili flakes

Directions:

1. Add cheese, chickpeas and spinach into a large bowl.

2. To make dressing: Add rest of the ingredients into another bowl and mix well.

3. Pour dressing over the salad. Toss well and serve.

Nutrition: Calories 822 Total Fat 42.5g Saturated Fat 11.7g Cholesterol 44mg Sodium 910mg Total Carbohydrate 89.6g Dietary Fiber 19.7g Total Sugars 32.7g Protein 29g Vitamin D 0mcg Calcium 417mg Iron 9mg Potassium 1347mg

Tempeh "Chicken" Salad

Preparation Time: 10 minutes

Cooking Time: 0 minutes

Servings: 2

Ingredients:

- 4 tablespoons light mayonnaise
- 2 scallions, sliced
- Pepper to taste
- 4 cups mixed salad greens
- 4 teaspoons white miso
- 2 tablespoons chopped fresh dill
- 1 ½ cups crumbled tempeh
- 1 cup sliced grape tomatoes

Directions:

To make dressing:

1. Add mayonnaise, scallions, miso, dill and pepper into a bowl and whisk well.
2. Add tempeh and fold gently.

To serve:

3. Divide the greens into 4 plates. Divide the tempeh among the plates. Top with tomatoes and serve.

Nutrition: Calories 452 Total Fat 24.5g Saturated Fat 4.4g Cholesterol 8mg Sodium 733mg Total Carbohydrate 37.2g Dietary Fiber 2.6g Total Sugars 5.3g Protein 29.9g Vitamin D 0mcg Calcium 261mg Iron 8mg Potassium 1377mg

Spinach & Dill Pasta Salad

Preparation Time: 5 minutes

Cooking Time: 0 minutes

Servings: 4

Ingredients:

For salad:

- 3 cups cooked whole-wheat fusilli
- 2 cups cherry tomatoes, halved
- ½ cup vegan cheese, shredded
- 4 cups spinach, chopped
- 2 cups edamame, thawed
- 1 large red onion, finely chopped

For dressing:

- 2 tablespoons white wine vinegar
- ½ teaspoon dried dill
- 2 tablespoons extra-virgin olive oil
- Salt to taste
- Pepper to taste

Directions:

To make dressing:

1. Add all the ingredients for dressing into a bowl and whisk well. Set aside for a while for the flavors to set in.

To make salad:

2. Add all the ingredients of the salad in a bowl. Toss well.
3. Drizzle dressing on top. Toss well.
4. Divide into 4 plates and serve.

Nutrition: Calories 684 Total Fat 33.6g Saturated Fat 4.6g Cholesterol 4mg Sodium 632mg Total Carbohydrate 69.5g Dietary Fiber 12g Total Sugars 6.4g Protein 31.7g Vitamin D 0mcg Calcium 368mg Iron 8mg Potassium 1241mg

Italian Veggie Salad

Preparation Time: 10 minutes

Cooking Time: 0 minutes

Servings: 8

Ingredients:

For salad:

- 1 cup fresh baby carrots, quartered lengthwise
- 1 celery rib, sliced
- 3 large mushrooms, thinly sliced
- 1 cup cauliflower florets, bite sized, blanched
- 1 cup broccoli florets, blanched
- 1 cup thinly sliced radish

Conclusion

Vegan recipes do not need to be boring. There are so many different combinations of veggies, fruits, whole grains, beans, seeds, and nuts that you will be able to make unique meal plans for many months. These recipes contain the instructions along with the necessary ingredients and nutritional information.

If you ever come across someone complaining that they can't follow the plant-based diet because it's expensive, hard to cater for, lacking in variety, or tasteless, feel free to have them take a look at this book. In no time, you'll have another companion walking beside you on this road to healthier eating and better living.

Although healthy, many people are still hesitant to give vegan food a try. They mistakenly believe that these would be boring, tasteless, and complicated to make. This is the farthest thing from the truth.

Fruits and vegetables are organically delicious, fragrant, and vibrantly colored. If you add herbs, mushrooms, and nuts to the mix, dishes will always come out packed full of flavor it only takes a bit of effort and time to prepare great-tasting vegan meals for your family.

How easy was that? Don't we all want a seamless and easy way to cook like this?

I believe cooking is taking a better turn and the days, when we needed so many ingredients to provide a decent meal, were gone. Now, with easy tweaks, we can make delicious, quick, and easy meals. Most importantly, we get to save a bunch of cash on groceries.

I am grateful for downloading this book and taking the time to read it. I know that you have learned a lot and you had a great time reading it. Writing books is the best way to share the skills I have with your and the best tips too.

I know that there are many books and choosing my book is amazing. I am thankful that you stopped and took time to decide. You made a great decision and I am sure that you enjoyed it.

I will be even happier if you will add some comments. Feedbacks helped by growing and they still do. They help me to choose better content and new ideas. So, maybe your feedback can trigger an idea for my next book.

Hopefully, this book has helped you understand that vegetarian recipes and diet can improve your life, not only by improving your health and helping you lose weight, but also by saving you money and time. I sincerely hope that the recipes provided in this book have proven to be quick, easy, and delicious, and have provided you with enough variety to keep your taste buds interested and curious.

I hope you enjoyed reading about my book!

Lightning Source UK Ltd.
Milton Keynes UK
UKHW021816160421
382089UK00001B/61